Published by
Adams Media Corporation
nter Street, Holbrook, MA 02343
www.adamsmedia.com

ISBN: 1-58062-427-8

Printed in Canada.

I H G F E D C B A

ongress Cataloging-in-Publication
on available from the publisher.

ed to provide accurate and authoritative informa-
bject matter covered. It is sold with the under-
r is not engaged in rendering legal, accounting,
ce. If legal advice or other expert assistance is
ompetent professional person should be sought.
ion of Principles jointly adopted by a Committee
American Bar Association and a Committee of
Publishers and Associations.

r photo by Superstock.

t quantity discounts for bulk purchases.
ion, call 1-800-872-5627.

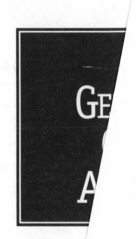

GE

C

A

CL

DISCLAIMER

This guide was written to offer options to the professional male. It should not be considered a guide to a strict code of dress. Following the advice in this booklet does not guarantee any specific benefits.

DEDICATION

This book is dedicated to my grandparents: Julie, Alex, Millie, and Clint. Thank you for your love, guidance, and support. I love you.

CONTENTS

PREFACE

This book began as a collection of notes that I wrote to help a few of my friends in college get an edge in job interviews. The idea was to help people who were smart and talented but needed some help with the basics of acting like a gentleman. Through no fault of their own, they had not been taught these rules and tricks of the trade. At a time when many young men do not know the rules of professional appearance and conduct, those who do have a clear advantage. The great news is that anyone can learn how to dress and act properly; this book will teach you how to do it.

I have received many letters from men who read earlier editions of this book and have thanked me for the extra boost of confidence they got from reading and referring to it before important interviews and meetings. The goal I had in writing this book was to provide you with information you will need to survive in the business world. I hope that everyone who reads this will be more confident once armed with the necessary information to dress and act professionally as a true gentleman.

INTRODUCTION

*Clothes make the man. Naked people have little
or no influence in society.* — Mark Twain

Let's face it, in today's world, appearance and conduct
matter. People are initially judged by the way they look.
They earn their credibility based on how they act.
Those who want to succeed take the time to look their
best and act appropriately for all occasions.

No matter your background, you can learn to look
great and conduct yourself like a professional by reading
this book. You will learn that attention to detail matters,
not only in your career, but in all aspects of your life.
The level of care reflected in your appearance and manners attracts positive attention and admiration, which
foster confidence. Most important, you will begin to pay
more attention to detail—a skill highly valued in the
professional world.

WHY APPEARANCE MATTERS 1

Who decided that tying some fabric around your neck will make you look more serious, or wearing shoes that are shined will give you the appearance of a go-getter? Research studies show that there is a high correlation between appearance and perceptions of professional abilities. Also, the first impression is the one that remains in most people's mind.

But the derivation and theories of societal grooming standards are not the point of this book, so it will not delve deeply into why it matters. As a reader, simply accept that it does. This book takes the stance that although individualism and self-expression are important, for most of us, dressing appropriately for the professional environment is necessary for success. This book is for those of you who wish to compete in today's professional world. While being well dressed is not enough to ensure success, an unprofessional appearance will almost guarantee failure. The point is not to tell you what you must do or wear, but to guide you in what is considered acceptable and preferred today. You will learn what it takes to display a professional image.

Shoes

Let us start with shoes. A great shine on your shoes can really enhance your professional image. The trick to a sparkling shoeshine is not elbow grease but technique. Once you have learned the technique, your shoes will stay shined and your overall appearance will be noticeably improved.

First, buy some shoe polish that matches your shoe color. Use black on black shoes, brown on brown shoes, and cordovan on oxblood shoes.

Place a few old newspapers on the floor before you start. You'll also need a cotton rag (an old T-shirt will do), a bit of water, and about 30 minutes per shoe (for the first time, 10 minutes after that). Separate each shoe into seven sections: (1) toe, (2) right front, (3) right back, (4) the heel, (5) left back, (6) left front, and (7) tongue (figure 1).

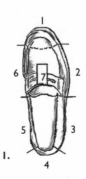

1.

Work on only one section at a time. Open the polish tin and fill the top cover with lukewarm water. Take your cloth rag and wrap it tightly around your right index and middle fingers (figure 2).

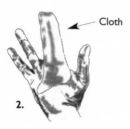

2.

Touch your fingers to the water in the lid, then smack them against your left palm to make sure the cloth is not too wet. Make a few circles in the polish with the moist rag. Now, using light pressure, make circles of polish on the first section of the shoe (figure 3).

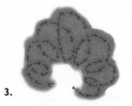

3.

Polish Motion

The trick here is to make small, tight circles as your fingers move around the section in a circular motion. As you apply the polish to your shoe, it will blur any existing shine. This means the polish is filling every pore in the leather. By moving in circles, you will compact the polish in each pore. Once all pores are filled with polish, a shine will become visible as light is reflected from the smooth, flat surface (figure 4).

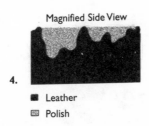

Magnified Side View

4.

■ Leather
▨ Polish

Once you have applied polish to the first section, move your fingers to a clean part of the rag. Wet it as described above. Using water only, make the same polishing motions with a little less pressure on the same section of the shoe. You should notice the beginning of a nice shine. This buffing action will further compact the polish and smooth it into the pores of the leather.

When you polish each shoe for the first time, repeat the process (starting with new polish and then buffing it in) three times per section. Once a week, reshine each section. This will take only about 10 minutes and will keep your shoes looking great.

Another way to make your shoes look their best is to use edge dressing. This is basically a paint, or dye, that coats the side of the sole. It seals and protects, as well as provides a finished look to your shoes. Several types are available, but Kiwi Honor Guard Edge Dressing is the best. Be careful with edge dressing, though, since it is a permanent dye and stains very easily. Remember to put newspaper on the floor, and apply the dressing only to the outer walls of the soles, not on the bottom. To fill the area where the leather meets the sole use a cotton swab to apply the edge dressing (figure 5). Be sure not to touch the leather. Once a week, touch up any areas that may have become scuffed, such as the toe and heel.

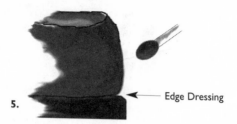

5. ←— Edge Dressing

After three or four months of constant wear and regular polishing, your shoes will become more difficult to shine. The polish will begin to build up in some areas and to crack and fall off. This leaves uneven layers of polish and a dull shine. To remedy this, you will need to break down the finish. This is a relatively simple but messy process, so again, lay down some newspaper. You will also need a few rags, a toothbrush, and a can of shaving cream, preferably the gel type.

First remove any laces from your shoes so they do not interfere with the process. If you have a gel-type shaving cream, spray it on your hand and make sure to work up a good lather. Rub it gently into the leather, covering it completely. After both shoes are covered with shaving cream, set them aside for about four hours to break down the chemical bonds of the polish and allow it to detach from the leather. At the same time, the cream will condition the shoe as it moisturizes and softens the leather.

After four hours have passed, take the rags and carefully wipe the cream off the shoes. You will notice that along with the cream, your rags will collect some old polish. Be sure to wipe the shaving cream off completely; if it stays on the shoe, it will flake off after you have repolished and will ruin the shine. Use the toothbrush to clean the shaving cream out of the small creases in the leather and the area where the sole meets the leather.

You should notice after breaking down the finish that the leather is more supple and has a duller shine. This is actually a good process for the shoe and can extend its useful life by as much as 50 percent.

The next step is to buy some shoe cream. It comes in a smaller jar than polish but is based on the same color scheme. First, cover the leather with the cream. Use a rag and the same polishing motion described above. After the cream covers the shoe, brush it in with a horsehair brush. If you don't have a brush, you can take a clean part of the rag and rub it into the leather. Let it sit for about an hour and the cream will get to work. Now simply repeat the process of shining as described in the beginning of this chapter.

You will also discover that your shoes will last two to three times longer than usual if you buy at least two pairs and alternate them daily (figure 6).

6.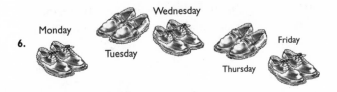

For example, if you have a black and a brown pair, you would wear the black on Monday, brown on Tuesday, black on Wednesday, etc.

When you shoes are not worn, cedar shoetrees will help them keep their form and allow them to dry and air out completely. Shoetrees are essentially molds of feet that you place in your shoes when you are not wearing them so that the shoes keep their shape. Without a shoetree, when you take off your shoes the leather will sink down and begin to shrink. The sweat from your feet soaks the leather and causes it to mold to the misformed shape.

A good shoetree will push the leather to its intended shape. It will also help dry the leather from your sweat and keep it from damaging and cracking the shoe. One other benefit of shoetrees is that they help reduce odor after the shoes are worn. Good quality shoetrees are made of cedar and absorb both sweat and odor before your next wearing. You can buy a cheap plastic pair for less than $10, but they are essentially useless. They are flimsy, hollow, and do not adjust well to your shoes.

The best shoetree on the market is the Woodlore model seen in figure 7. It has a split toe that expands to fit the width of the shoe and an overhang heel for easy removal.

7.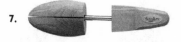

You can find Woodlore shoetrees at fine men's stores or on the Web at www.greenleafenterprises.com.

If you are in a professional office environment, be sure to buy leather-soled shoes. Leather-soled shoes have a certain quality about them that rubber-soled shoes do not have. The marginal improvement in comfort you see with rubber soles will not replace the loss of credibility you will incur by wearing rubber soles.

During the winter months, the high level of salt used to melt snow on the ground will, invariably, get on your shoes. Often, this salt accumulates on leather shoes and wreaks havoc with a good shine and your leather. The white stain is almost impossible to get off, but worse, the salt will destroy your shoes.

The best way to remove this salt is a 50-50 mixture of water and white vinegar. Mix the two in the top of a shoe polish tin. Dab a clean rag in the mixture and rub it into the salt lines of the shoe. After it looks like you have removed it, allow it to dry for about 20 minutes. Check to be sure all of it is removed. If not, simply repeat the process.

Once all the salt is removed, apply some shoe cream to the treated area and polish it as usual.

A good shine and a few well cared for pairs of leather-soled shoes will clearly illustrate your attention to detail and professionalism. This is an extremely easy way to show others that you care about your appearance and increase your credibility.

SHIRTS

Although casual Fridays allow us to relax our style of dress once a week, chances are you need to wear a dress shirt to work most of the time. A pressed dress shirt shows that you care about your appearance and helps you look more fit. Have your shirts professionally washed and ironed. It may seem like an unnecessary expense, but the benefits are more than worth it. For less than two dollars a day, your shirts will be ironed properly. If you check around you may find dry cleaners who will pick up and deliver directly to your door.

For those times when you realize that you have to iron your shirt and you cannot find a 24-hour cleaner, however, here are the basic steps. The only tools you'll need are an iron and an ironing board. If, for some reason, you do not have an iron, your best (and only) bet is to turn on the shower as hot as possible, hang your shirt in the bathroom, and close the door. This will steam your shirt and take out some of the wrinkles. If you are staying at a hotel, check for an iron and ironing board; there should be one in your closet or at the front desk. If you have an iron and not the board, get a thick towel and place it on any hard surface.

Check the tag on your shirt to make sure that the fabric can handle steam ironing. Now, pour some distilled water into the iron. If it does not have a hole on top, get a spray bottle and fill it with water. To make the job easier, keep the fabric lightly damp.

The first part is the collar, and it is quite important. Flatten the collar and move from the points to the back of the neck on both sides. Take extra care to be sure that the points are straight.

To smooth out the shoulder, place it on the corner of the board or table to simulate your shoulder. Place the sleeves onto the ironing board or table and iron each sleeve on both sides. Mist the fabric and place the iron at the cuff. Pull the iron from the shoulder seam to the cuff.

From the shoulder, move to the front of your shirt and start on the side with buttons. Stretch it out and move the iron from the shoulder down to the bottom. Be careful when you iron between the buttons; it is easy to melt or snap them. Now iron the back of the shirt; again, iron from the shoulder to the bottom. You can now finish off on the other front half of the shirt.

A properly pressed shirt must be tucked in well. After you button it, gently pull down and out on the front of the shirt (figure 8). This will straighten the button line so it is directly in the middle of your body. Now, slide your hands around your sides from your front to your back to bunch any loose cloth in the back (figure 9).

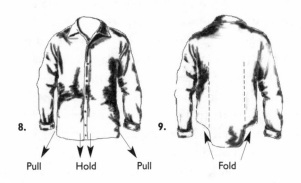

8.

Pull   Hold   Pull

9.

Fold

Take the excess in your hands and fold it over toward the outside. Holding your shirt in position, pull up your pants and lock the shirt in place. This trick will keep your front free of wrinkles and folds, and the fold in the back will nicely hide any excess fabric (figure 10).

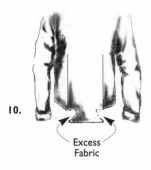

10.

Excess
Fabric

When you buy your shirts be sure that the material is opaque. It is not appropriate to see chest hair or a T-shirt through the fabric. Also, wear only long-sleeved shirts with a suit. If you feel the need to have shorter sleeves, you can always roll them up.

A T-shirt should be worn underneath most dress shirts, even in the summer. The T-shirt should have a full neck and short sleeves. V-necks and tank tops are visible under most dress shirts and look inappropriate. Wearing a T-shirt may make you a little warmer, but deal with the heat and cover yourself; it does matter.

Many shirts have collars and cuffs made from a contrasting color, for example a blue shirt with white collar and cuffs. These shirts come in and out of style and are acceptable only in certain circles. A good rule is to watch what other people in your office wear, and how certain styles are received. If your office is stylish, feel free to wear such a shirt. If your office is very conservative, you may wish to keep your shirts a solid color. By keeping an eye on the general attire of the office, you demonstrate that you are paying attention to detail and enhancing your professional appearance.

Several types of shirt collars are available. There are four basic types: the button-down collar, the point collar, the snap-tab collar, and the sculptured collar (figure 11). Each type is considered appropriate for business. The right choice depends on personal taste. One word of caution though: If you wear button-down collars, make sure that both sides are buttoned. If your collars are not buttoned down, get your cleaner to heavily starch your collars. The starch will keep your collar from curling up and looking unprofessional. Remember that your image is always under scrutiny.

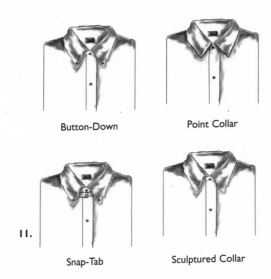

Button-Down   Point Collar

II.

Snap-Tab   Sculptured Collar

Men often wonder about the merits of purchasing custom-made shirts versus ready-made shirts. Essentially, off-the-rack shirts are fine if they fit you well. If your frame is unique, and you find it difficult to find shirts that fit, custom shirts may be for you. Some men consider custom-made shirts superior, but the great majority wear off-the-rack clothes and still look professional.

TIES 4

Almost every professional man must wear a tie. Unfortunately, 80 percent look sloppy. This is often the result of a half-Windsor knot (also known as the four-in-hand), which makes ties appear asymmetrical. A poll of executives revealed that most believe a half-Windsor knot looks unprofessional, and a double-Windsor knot looks too bulky. The survey concluded that a full-Windsor looks best for business (figure 12).

12.

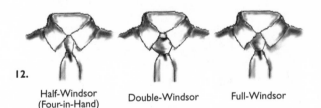

Half-Windsor   Double-Windsor   Full-Windsor
(Four-in-Hand)

To tie a full-Windsor knot, put your tie around your neck with the wide base on the left and the thin end on the right. Pull the tie so that the bottom of the thin section is even with the third button down from the top of your shirt (figure 13). Now pull the wide section over the thin section, making an X (figure 14). With your left hand, reach under the X and pull the wide section under, then over the upper left part of the X (figure 15). Pull the wide section through the upper half of the X, then through so it points toward the ground (figure 16). Now turn the wide section to the right side, then over the center of the tie to the left side of the X (figure 17). Pull the wide section up through the back side of the upper half of the X (figure 18). Make sure to leave a bit of slack on the front as you pull the wide section through the cross you just made (figure 19). You've done it!

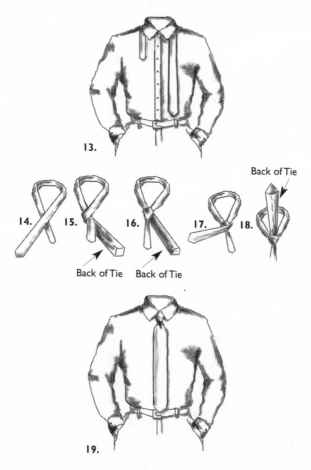

Back of Tie

13.

14.   15.   16.   17.   18.

Back of Tie   Back of Tie

19.

The first few times you use this method you might have a little bit of trouble getting it to sit properly. The wide part should be longer than the thin part, and the tip of the wide part should be even with the bottom of your belt buckle. Be sure that the bottom of the tie does not end above your buckle or extend too far below the belt. Do not worry if you are not right on the first few tries, over time it will become second nature.

Although prevalent through the 1960s, tie clips and tiepins are no longer in style. If your tie is properly tied, it will remain in place without a clip or pin. However, if you want to wear a clip or pin with your suit, feel free. Simply understand that it conveys an older image.

Most men only wear bow ties with tuxedos, but learning how to tie a bow tie is considered an art. To learn the art of tying a bow tie, follow the example below: the tie we will use is half white, half black, as seen in figure 20.

Begin by wrapping the white end around the middle of the black side, and pull the ends out to the side, much like the first step of tying a shoe (figure 21). Now take the white end, and fold it three ways as seen in the diagram (figure 22). This will form the front of the bow, a sort of a T. Press the white bow against your throat, and wrap the black piece over the front, middle, of the tie (figure 23). Make the same kind of three-fold T with the end of the black piece. Now, pull the black bow behind the white bow and between the fabric closest to your neck and the white bow (figure 24). You should end up with two bows, the white in front, and the black in back (figure 25). Now pull gently on the bows to tighten the knot, and you have a formal bow tie!

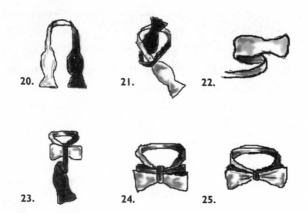

20.   **21.**   **22.**

23.   **24.**   **25.**

Although you may not have many opportunities to wear one, the ability to tie a real bow tie will add credibility to your character. Few men know how. While bow ties are not recommended for daily wear, some professionals make it their style. Professionally speaking, however, bow ties are definitely not mainstream, and possibly the mark of an eccentric.

PANTS 5

Wearing pants seems easy enough, right? While pants are not nearly as problematic as ties or shirts, pants do require a bit of care. In the professional world, you will spend most of your time sitting, which causes your pants to wear faster than your jacket. This will create a mismatch in color and quality between your jacket and pants, which looks quite unprofessional. Although it is somewhat inevitable, there are steps you can take to slow the process.

Carry your wallet in the breast pocket of your jacket instead of your pants to prevent your pant pocket from wearing out. Another option is to carry a money clip for your bills and a cardholder for your credit cards and driver's license. If you put one in each front pant pocket, you will be able to carry your valuables with you without seriously damaging your pockets.

Keys and coins are another pocket killer. If you must carry keys, limit them to only the ones you must have to make it through the workday. Both keys and coins will leave outlines on your pants or make holes in your pockets if they are carried in the same pocket day after day. It is considered unprofessional to walk with coins and keys "clinking" around in your pocket, so limit the amount of coins you have and keep them in a different pocket than your keys.

When you remove your suit after the workday is over, folding your pants properly will ensure a good crease and fewer wrinkles. Begin by holding your pants upside down and lining up all four seams (figure 26). Pull the front and back of the pant out at the cuff, keeping the seams together. The fold should fall on the natural crease of the pants. Slip the pants onto a hanger, replace the jacket, and hang it up in your closet.

When wrinkles become noticeable, pressing your pants becomes an important part of keeping a professional appearance. Pressed pants will make your suit look sharper and illustrate your attention to detail. The good news is that pressing your pants does not necessarily mean dry-cleaning them. You can press them with an iron in about a minute and bring your pants back to life. Before you do, however, make sure to check the care label in your suit to be sure the material can be ironed.

Line up the seams of your pants as detailed above, lay them on an ironing table, and press out the wrinkles. Depending on the fabric, consider using a pressing cloth or turning the pants inside out to avoid burning or a shiny surface to your pants. Either will look extremely unprofessional.

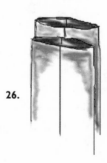

26.

The "Gig-Line" 6

As you get ready to buckle your belt, look at your shirt. Your "gig-line" should be straight. The gig-line is a vertical line that runs the length of your body from your zipper to your collar. This line has three major components: pants, belt, and shirt. The right side of your zipper should be even with the button on the top of your pants. Use this as your guide. Next, take the button line of your shirt and pull it down so that the right edge of the line is even with your zipper line. The third part requires you to pull the belt so that the right edge of your buckle is even with your pant and shirt line. Your tie will follow the gig-line naturally and end up at the bottom of your belt buckle. This is a straight gig-line, and it really makes a difference in overall professional appearance (figure 27).

Gig-Line

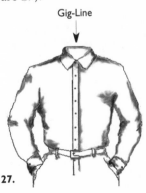

27.

Jackets

The key to finding the right jacket is to buy a high-quality suit that fits your frame, is well tailored, and is a basic color. Although some businessmen remove their suit jackets during the day, the jacket is an integral part of the professional wardrobe. Make sure to hang up your jacket when you are not wearing it, especially when you are driving to work. While sitting at your desk, remove your jacket if you can. Make sure you keep extra hangers in your office. When you wear your jacket, button only the top button. Walking with an open jacket looks sloppy, and buttoning two buttons looks too rigid. When you sit down while wearing a jacket, be sure to unbutton it. If you are interested in a classy look, consider a pocket handkerchief that matches your tie.

A jacket that fits properly is the most basic item in your professional attire. It is, however, not cheap. Again, as with all clothing, paying for quality is the best way to go. First, find the style of suit best fitted for your frame. There are three main styles: athletic, regular, and full. If you have a typical American male frame, you will probably wear a regular-style suit. If you are in great shape, the athletic style may be the best. If you have a more portly figure, try the full cut.

To find the right sleeve length, stretch your arms out in front of you. The edge of the sleeve should touch the wrist bone that sticks up on the outside of your arm. Fitting the shirt should be a similar process. The shirt should extend a half-inch beyond the edge of the jacket when your arms are outstretched (figure 28).

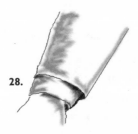

28.

To get the right jacket length, stand with your hands straight down and your fingers curled as if to hold a pencil. The jacket bottom should just touch your fingers where the pencil would set.

Buy the highest-quality suit that looks good on you and that you can afford. Single-breasted suits are more common in the professional world than double-breasted suits, but feel free to go with the look you prefer. The basic colors are navy blue and charcoal gray. Olive green and light gray are also acceptable in some professions.

Once you have purchased the right suit, you must prepare it before you wear it. Go to a qualified tailor and
have your suits altered to fit your body. When your suit
is back from the tailor, search for small pieces of loose
thread improperly cut in the factory or by the tailor.
These little strings are sometimes referred to
euphemistically as "pendants." Good hiding places for
the threads are near buttons, buttonholes, and on and
near seams (figure 29). Clip the threads as close to the
body of the fabric as possible with nail clippers.

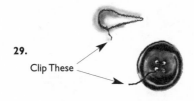

29.

Clip These

BUYING SUITS 8

When you buy suits, you need to be prepared. You have to go into the store armed with good information and an understanding of what you want. First, know which of the three basic suit cuts will fit you best (figure 30).

These are the three basic body types that will help you determine the proper cut of suit to purchase.

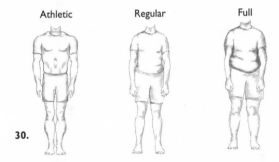

Athletic   Regular   Full

30.

You should also consider the purpose of the suit. Is it for work in a professional environment, or is it for more casual affairs? This should also be part of the decision of the type of suit you purchase.

When you buy suits, you first choose the right jacket size; the average American male is about a 42. The "drop" is the difference from jacket size to pant waist. Most suits have a drop of seven inches, so a 42 suit will come with a 35-inch waist.

The vent is the slit in the back of the suit that is usually about six inches long. The purpose of the vent is to allow a man with a larger bottom to fit into a suit in which the shoulders are not very wide. For example, a pear-shaped man would want to wear a suit with vents, but a chiseled Marine has little need for vents.

As a general rule, full suits have two vents, regulars have one, and athletic suits have none. If you have a large backside, you should consider a suit with at least one vent.

The question of a single- or double-breasted suit is common, and it is really a matter of personal preference. If you like a broad-chested look, then a double-breasted suit is right for you. Although double-breasted suits are considered more formal, they are less common in the professional workplace. If you do wear a double-breasted suit, remember to keep it buttoned at all times.

There are two basic choices with your pants: pleats and cuffs. A pleat is the fold in the pants just below the belt line between the zipper and the pocket. The standard for professional suit pants is a double pleat. Make sure that the pleats lay flat and are not pulled apart. If they are pulled apart, this is a sign that you need wider pants.

Most suit pants are sold with cuffs, and they are considered standard on dress pants. Unless you have a good reason not to like cuffs, be sure to get them on your next pair of suit pants.

Finally, when purchasing a suit, be sure to bring a close and honest friend along with you to give you some useful feedback on the fit of the suits. Try on several different styles and sizes and do not skimp on quality. As soon as you purchase your suits, take them to a reputable tailor and have the suits tailored to fit you perfectly.

FORMAL WEAR 9

While many professionals do not need to wear formal wear, the formal party is still part of many businesses. This simple description will give you the basic information you need to attend formal parties with confidence.

A tuxedo has pants, a pleated shirt, a bow tie, a jacket, and either a cummerbund or a vest. Tails, on the other hand, are considered more formal. They are similar to a tuxedo, but have a jacket that extends well below the waist; hence the term "tails." They do not have cummerbunds but do have a white tie and white vest.

When you see the phrase "Black-Tie Optional" on an invitation, it usually means that you can wear either a suit or a tuxedo. To save yourself from the embarrassment of underdressing, use this as a chance to wear your tuxedo.

The phrase "Black-Tie Optional" used to mean that a man had the option to wear a tuxedo or tails.

For most young men, it makes sense to rent tuxedos through their high school years. As a general rule, as soon as you stop growing, you should consider buying your own tuxedo. If you are often invited to very formal events, consider also purchasing a tails jacket.

If you buy a tuxedo, be sure to have it tailored so that it fits you well. You will look terrible wearing formal wear if it is poorly tailored. Also, buy two or three tuxedo shirts with pleats; your usual dress shirt will not work.

Whether you are buying or renting, make sure the jacket and pants are black. You can be as colorful as you want to be with your tie and cummerbund, but colored tuxedos are just not appropriate. This black rule continues with your feet as well. Your socks and your shoes should both be black. If your usual dress black shoes are well shined, you might be able to wear them with your tux. However, you might consider buying a patent leather pair only for your tuxedo.

Studs, the little knobs that go in the buttonholes on your shirt, are usually appropriate. The cummerbund is the large belt-like object that wraps around your waist. Make sure to wear it with the folds facing up. If you have a large stomach, do not try to wear a cummerbund; wear a vest.

Many professionals choose not to attend formal functions because they do not know how to dress properly. Do not limit your career simply because of a lack of information.

CLEANING YOUR CLOTHES 10

Stains and spots on your clothes are a fact of life. What follows is a general guide on what you can use to remove certain spots.

Aside from being quite annoying, paper cuts can go undetected until blood appears on your shirt. As soon as you notice a blood stain, blot it with a paper towel. Then run the fabric under cold water for a few minutes. At the earliest possible convenience, wash the fabric with color-safe bleach.

Deodorant stains should be blotted with white vinegar, then the fabric washed with a color-safe bleach in the hottest water allowable (check the label for the recommended temperature). An old perspiration stain that has caused the fabric to yellow should also be blotted with white vinegar. Fresh perspiration stains may be blotted with ammonia water (one teaspoon per quart). After blotting, soak the fabric in cold water, then wash it in the hottest water allowable for the fabric.

During the working day, other stains can occur. In general, most stains can be cleaned by blotting—not rubbing—then soaking the fabric in cold water. When you wash your clothes, use color-safe bleach. Black coffee stains can be treated in this manner, as can stains from chocolate, fruit juices, and soft drinks. Ink from a ballpoint pen can be removed from fabric with hairspray. Simply spray the spot, let it soak into the fabric, then wash the garment with color-safe bleach.

In caring for your clothes, again, you must be willing to pay the price necessary to keep your appearance impeccable. If you tend to be thrifty, you might be tempted to wear your shirts two or three times before getting them cleaned. Don't do it. Pay the extra money to wear a clean shirt every day. Wrinkles and spots will destroy not only your appearance but your credibility as a professional as well.

On the other hand, there is no set rule for how often you must clean your suits. The Neighborhood Cleaning Association (an action group of dry cleaners) suggests cleaning after one to three wearings. Others say you can wait up to 12 wearings. As a general rule, you can wear your suits until you feel they are dirty and need to be cleaned. This usually means about 5 to 10 wearings, but make sure you feel comfortable with the cleanliness of your wardrobe. When you dry-clean your suits, have the pants and jacket done together to ensure that the color continues to match.

ACCESSORIES 11

Now that your clothes are set, you need accessories. For starters, you need a business watch. This is a watch that looks professional with your suits, but is not too flashy. As a general rule, leather and metal bands (gold, silver, and stainless steel) are advisable. Avoid digital faces and plastic bands. Another important accessory is a leather belt. You will need one black belt and one brown belt, or a single convertible belt, with a nice silver or gold buckle. Remember, though, that you are not a cowboy, so keep the buckle size small.

Many professionals look great wearing braces, also called suspenders. Suspenders are a substitute for a belt, so wear one or the other but not both. The key to wearing suspenders properly is to pay to have buttons sewn into your pants to anchor the straps. No self-respecting professional (or even clown) wears clip-on suspenders. The color of your suspenders should match your tie. As usual, choosing a solid color or basic pattern makes matching much easier. Also remember that out-landish colors may not be appropriate.

Buy a high-quality pen and avoid carrying a cheap pen during any interview or meeting. You can find a nice pen for about $10, but don't be afraid to pay for quality. A prestigious pen will really make you look good, just as a cheap pen can take away from your professional appearance.

Mont Blanc, Waterman, and Cross are among the premiere manufacturers of high-quality pens.

Along with the pen, it is advisable to carry a leather-bound portfolio for important documents and your business cards. You can buy a generic portfolio or carry one from your school or company. The idea is to carry loose papers in a professional looking way at all times. If you find a need to carry several items, a leather or metal briefcase can be a fine accessory. Make sure, however, that it looks professional and not like an old gym bag.

Cologne should be used sparingly since people are turned off by an overpowering scent. As a general rule, use about half the amount you would use if you were going on a date. Put it on about fifteen minutes before you leave your house, as it takes a few minutes to dissipate. Use it to enhance your appearance, not dominate it.

Clean hands are imperative in business. While a manicure might not be necessary (although many businessmen do get weekly manicures), it is important to keep your hands and fingernails clean. Your fingernails should be trimmed (not bitten) cleanly just past the quick. This will give you about $1/16$ of an inch of white at the end of each nail.

To always look your best, consider keeping an extra dress shirt, tie, and umbrella in your office or car. At some point, a stain on your shirt or tie is inevitable. Having an extra shirt and tie handy will add a level of security to your professional appearance. The extra umbrella will keep your suit dry; a hard rain can really ruin a suit. Also, keep a few toothpicks in your car and briefcase. Few things are as embarrassing as belatedly noticing that you have part of your last meal in your teeth.

Be very careful about wearing any jewelry besides a watch. Wedding rings and, in some cases, college and military rings are acceptable. Bracelets, necklaces, and some rings, however, are not. Earrings, nose rings, eyebrow rings, and other body piercing jewelry are generally taboo. Excessive jewelry is considered inappropriate. Now that the 1970s are well behind us, necklaces and bracelets in the workplace are too. Tattoos are usually not acceptable in a professional environment. If you have one, keep it covered.

The handkerchief used to be an integral part of the male wardrobe but has, in recent years, become much less popular. The two reasons for still wearing a handkerchief are for function, instead of tissues, and for fashion, in your coat pocket. It does provide a professional look, but be sure to fold it so that a triangle shows out of the pocket (figure 31).

Folding a Handkerchief

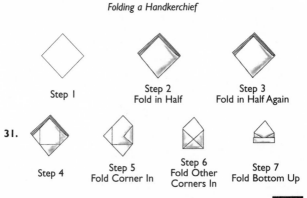

31.

Step 1

Step 2
Fold in Half

Step 3
Fold in Half Again

Step 4

Step 5
Fold Corner In

Step 6
Fold Other Corners In

Step 7
Fold Bottom Up

Another valuable accessory is a lint roller, which is a rod with a cylinder of double-sided tape on the end of it. You roll it over your clothes to pick up small pieces of lint, dirt, hair, and other undesirable debris. If you have pets, you must use a lint roller. Because they are so cheap, you can keep several around for your convenience.

There is an unwritten code at many companies that facial hair gives a bad first impression. If you choose to wear a beard or mustache, check with those in your office to be sure that it is not frowned upon.

Assuming you do not have a beard or mustache, you must shave every day. There are no exceptions. Stubble can make you look like a teenager or a miscreant instead of a professional, no matter how well you dress.

There is a right way to shave, and unfortunately, most men just do not know how to do it. It is most important to shave with the grain initially. The following illustrations show how to shave with the grain.

Start with a downstroke from the sideburn to the jawbone (figure 32). From there, continue the downstroke from the jawline to the mid-neck. Note that you stop mid-neck, right around your Adam's apple (figure 33).

32.   **33.**

Most men make the mistake of continuing the down-stroke past the mid-neck; the problem with this is that the grain of the hair grows up from the lower neck to the mid-neck. So shave from the bottom of your neck to your Adam's apple. Next, shave straight down from your nose to your upper lip. Use sidestrokes to shave from the upper lip to the cheek.

There are several different kinds of shaving cream, but the two basic types are foamy and gel. The gel is a bit more expensive but usually provides a cleaner shave with less irritation. You might also consider several of the after-shave products. They might burn a bit on contact but will seal small nicks and provide a fresh scent.

If you find after shaving this way that you still need to remove more hair, repeat the process above, this time going across, then against, the grain of your face. Realize, however, that shaving across or against the grain will further irritate your skin.

SEWING ON BUTTONS 13

Another key to maintaining your wardrobe is a rudimentary knowledge of sewing. This doesn't mean you have to make your own clothes, but having the ability to sew a button back on your shirt is important. You will need a needle, about two feet of thread, and a button. You can buy these supplies cheaply at almost any store; it's a good idea to keep a small sewing kit in your briefcase or car just to be safe.

The color of thread should match the original color used by the manufacturer. If you cannot get a close match, though, use a neutral color that will not attract attention to the button.

Begin by threading the needle. Bring the two ends of the thread together and tie a triple knot. Now take the button and place it where the old button had been; there should be an indentation on the fabric.

Begin underneath the button side of the fabric, and push the needle through the fabric and into hole A (figure 34). Pull the needle through the hole until the knot is pulled tightly against the underside of the fabric. Each time you pull the needle through a hole and fabric, be sure to pull it completely through to eliminate any slack in the thread. Now push the needle through hole B into the fabric. From the underside, pull the needle through the fabric and push up into hole D. Next, place the needle into hole C and push through the fabric, remembering to pull the thread taut. This will hold the button in place and allow you to secure it for the actual sewing.

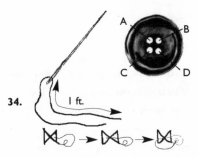

Now you can pull the needle through the fabric into hole A, into hole B, and back into the fabric. Return to hole A and repeat the process four times. After the fourth time through hole B, push the needle up through the fabric and into hole D. Push the needle through hole C, into the fabric, and back up through hole D. Repeat this four times.

Now that you're on the underside of the fabric, you'll need to tie off the thread. To do this, pull the needle underneath the developed knot, capturing a thread or two of the fabric. As you pull it through, leave a small loop at the other side. Pull the needle back through the loop and pull the thread taut.

Repeat this with another loop. Now, simply cut the thread just above the knot. With your button in place, you will easily maintain your wardrobe, saving you countless trips to the tailor.

MIXING AND MATCHING 14

Matching is a difficult prospect for most men. The key is to stick to the basics unless you have great style. If you think you have great style, this guide will help reaffirm your basic knowledge. For those of you whose inability to match may severely limit your success, here are some basic guidelines.

The key element to a simple matching wardrobe is a white shirt, so begin with about eight. They are easiest to match with a tie and suit. Next, buy at least one charcoal gray and one navy blue suit and two pairs of black shoes. The key to your simple wardrobe—and to disguising the fact that it is a simple wardrobe—is a variety of ties. You need about ten ties, in basic designs such as paisleys, solids, simple stripes, and small patterns. Red, maroon, and yellow ties are considered power colors, and complement both suit colors. Dark blue, royal blue, and green ties go well with gray but not with navy. Black socks are the best bet, especially if you are wearing black shoes. Never wear socks that are darker than your shoes. If you wish, you can match your socks to the dark colors in your tie. Your socks (and pants) should be long enough so that when you cross your legs, no skin shows.

Building your wardrobe to a slightly more advanced level is not difficult. Try a gray suit with black shoes, a solid blue shirt, and a yellow tie. Another good combination is an olive suit with maroon (cordovan) shoes, white shirt, and a multicolored tie with some olive in it. You may also consider a light gray suit, white shirt, red tie, and black shoes. These combinations will spice up your professional appearance.

BUSINESS CASUAL 15

Almost everyone loves casual Fridays, but what does "casual" really mean in the workplace? Unfortunately, there is no universal definition. As a general guide, if you are at all unsure about how casual you can be, do not guess. Wear appropriate professional clothing on the first casual day and observe what your coworkers wear. Depending on your type of business, the weather, your city, and the standards of casual dressing in your office, what is considered casual may vary greatly.

Khakis or dark dress pants are generally acceptable everywhere. With a button-down dress shirt, you can fit into almost any casual workplace. When weather permits, a golf or polo shirt may be acceptable; jeans often are not, so check with your coworkers before you risk it. Hats are never appropriate, nor are T-shirts or shorts. You can wear boat shoes, loafers, or even your usual dress shoes if they match the rest of your clothes. In the winter, a sweater is a good idea. Be sure to wear a collared shirt underneath the sweater, though. Remember, you do have coworkers, so do not forgo socks.

In America, a great deal of business is done on the golf course, and some companies are even paying for lessons for their employees to learn to play golf. (Incidentally, note that one "plays golf" and does not "go golf*ing*." Golf is a noun like tennis, not a verb like swim.)

When playing golf for business, unless you are in a throwback tournament, you will not need to wear a suit to the course. The suggested clothing for an afternoon of golf would be a collared shirt with long pants or possibly shorts, depending on the weather. Your shirt may be any color, but it should be clean and match your pants. Usually, your best bet is khaki-colored pants or shorts.

Some companies are now instituting "business ready" policies. Business ready is a modified form of business casual that requires you to have a jacket and tie ready, just in case a client visits or a surprise meeting is called. It is always a good idea to be ready to dress up if the circumstances demand it.

CLOTHES CHECKLIST 16

Here is a summary of the clothes you should have in your professional wardrobe:

Items	Quantity	Description
Suits	2–6	At least one charcoal gray and one navy blue to start
Dress Shirts	12+	Broken down as follows:
White	8	
Solid Color	2	Blue, pink
Striped	2	Blue with white and maroon with white
Ties	10	Conservative, not "fun" ties
Dress shoes	2–3	Black pair, brown pair
Dress belts	2	One black and one brown or a single convertible
Socks	18	10 black; 4 brown/khaki; 4 other colors/designs
Raincoat	1	
Accessories		
Watch	1	High quality
Umbrellas	2	One in the car, one in the office
Quality pen	1	Names like Mont Blanc, Waterman, or Cross

If you have these items, you will dress like a professional gentleman. Remember, high-quality clothes and accessories will help you look great with much less effort.

PHYSICAL FITNESS 17

A discussion of professional appearance would be incomplete without at least mentioning the benefits of staying, or getting, in shape. Although there are successful professionals who succeed without being in shape, many truly successful businessmen are in great shape. They spend the time to work out and tone their bodies. They also have more stamina and are able to more easily deal with working long hours. It is easier to fit into your clothes, you will have more energy, and you will look like a mover and shaker.

This chapter will not go into all the health benefits you can get from being in shape—but it is proven that you will live longer and better, sleep better, and have a better chance of beating a serious illness if you are in shape. This chapter also will not discuss the benefits for your personal relationships if you are in shape. Never mind that your significant other will probably find you more attractive and be happier with your "in shape" body. If you are single, imagine the ways that you will be more marketable if you are in shape.

So why should you care? Your professional career is predicated on your ability to deal with things like stress and pressure, long hours, and the occasional sprint through the airport to catch a flight. A good routine that includes stretching, a cardiovascular workout (running or swimming), and strength training will help you increase your stamina for those long nights at the office. When you finally get home, being in shape will help you fall asleep faster and more soundly.

Strength training will help you lose weight: it takes more than ten times as many calories to maintain one pound of muscle as it does one pound of fat.

Pressure at the office will seem much less overwhelming if you can keep in shape; somehow an overdue report isn't as daunting if you just made it through a four-mile hill run that morning. And then there is always the increased confidence that comes from looking your best. Not arrogance, but a more subtle form of confidence that is pervasive in the business world. People often do business with those who are confident and enthusiastic. Why not use this to your advantage and look your best?

This does not mean that your career depends on four hours a day in the gym. By taking about one hour every other day to exercise, you can trim down, keep your heart healthy, and have more energy. After consulting with your doctor, establish a workout plan. Decide the time of day you will work out and what you will do. Allow about an hour for your workout, plus time to cool down and have a shower afterward. If you do this every other day for a month, you will see a positive change in your professional appearance.

After you work out, make sure to take care of your body by drinking water. A gallon of water a day is recommended. This may sound like a lot, but water is the most important component of your body. Refresh it, and you will stay healthy and in shape. Instead of eating three meals a day, try eating only when you are hungry, even if that means six or seven times a day. Eat just until you are no longer hungry, not until you are full. This will raise your metabolism, allowing you to burn fat at a more rapid rate.

POSTURE 18

Good posture is an important part of your appearance. The way you sit, stand, and walk are all interpreted by others as keys to your attitude, strength, and ability to accomplish difficult tasks. Go-getters sit up straight, stand with style, and walk tall. So, how should you carry yourself?

When sitting down, sit as if you have strings attached to your chest and shoulders. Imagine that the string is pulling you up, so that you sit up straight. This will allow you to think more clearly, feel more energetic, and look professional.

When standing, fight the urge to put your hands in your pockets, fold your arms, or move your hands. If you are constantly fidgeting, you will attract attention away from your words. The most professional way to stand when waiting or speaking with someone is with your hands at your sides in a relaxed position. This conveys your willingness to listen, your patience and professionalism.

You can really take away from your own credibility by walking hunched over. When you are walking, imagine that the strings that were attached to your chest and shoulders are now moving with you, keeping your shoulders and head straight and your chin up. Smile when you walk, even if you live in New York City. When you grimace, you appear angry; smiling also helps improve your attitude.

CHIVALRY 19

Those who say chivalry is dead are wrong. Those who say chivalry is chauvinistic are also wrong. A true gentleman treats both men and women with respect. When you get to a door first, hold it open for others before you enter yourself. After you have gone through it, look behind to see if you could hold it for someone else. When entering an elevator, wait for all people exiting to leave, then hold the door for anyone waiting. When you reach your floor, hold the door for anyone who wants to enter. When at a table with a woman, take her coat and push in her chair.

When you are walking down the street with a woman, take the position on the outside, closest to the cars. This is considered old-fashioned but extremely classy. Although the pragmatic need to stand on the outside is considerably lessened in this modern era of paved streets, any observant person will see the gentlemanly nature of your acts and be impressed that you know how to treat people properly.

When entering a car, open the woman's door first, then you may enter. Remember that the most senior person should sit in the most comfortable seat, usually in the front. It is a good rule to be the last one in the car, especially if you are driving.

The concepts of chivalry and gender equality are not mutually exclusive. A true gentleman knows that by being chivalrous he is simply being kind and considerate, not asserting his dominance.

BUSINESS ETIQUETTE 20

In the business world, proper etiquette is a must. Those who do not follow the rules of accepted behavior, lose; it is as simple as that. Although this book is not long enough to discuss every aspect of proper etiquette, what follows is a rudimentary guide to selected important aspects.

> For more information on business etiquette, refer to my book Attention to Detail: A Gentleman's Guide to Professional Appearance and Conduct *(Greenleaf Enterprises, 1998).*

Proper appearance is part of proper etiquette. The other major aspect is demeanor, or what you say and how you act in a professional setting. Obvious points include avoiding emotional topics (such as religion and politics), and using Standard English when speaking (no slang, jargon, or vernacular).

Also keep in mind that seemingly insignificant aspects like good posture and a calm smile give the appearance of strength and a positive attitude. While others may not consciously notice, studies show that people react more favorably to those with good posture and a smile. Notice that a calm smile is key, not a wide, goofy grin. A calm smile exudes dignity and power and is proven to relax others around you.

When walking with coworkers, be courteous. If you walk unusually slow or fast, adjust your speed to accommodate the others in your group. If you have a kitchen or coffee station in your office, do not be afraid to make coffee. Clean up after yourself. Spend an extra three minutes to clean up a mess or wash a dish or two, and you will generate an amazing amount of goodwill.

A business card is key to establishing yourself in the professional world. Hand them out to your friends, family, new and old acquaintances, and those who you feel may benefit you in the future. Also remember to ask for others' cards and save them; building a large file of cards can really pay off in the future. Keep in mind, however, that it is usually inappropriate for a junior person to ask a senior person for a card. Feel free to give your card in return, but make sure the senior person initiates the process.

When you get a card, jot a few notes on the back about how you met the person, issues you discussed, and personal information that you have in common. Keep the cards in a centralized location like a planner or a special three-ring binder with custom sheets that hold business cards. Contact the people at least once a year to keep the lines of communication open. Many people send a holiday card to everyone on their list; the marginal cost can help to build your professional image and create a powerful personal network.

In the past few years, the incredible proliferation of new mobile phone options has left us with many questions of etiquette. We've all seen rude people babbling on their cell phones in public places, from restaurants to public transportation, even in movie theaters. This new technology went mainstream before we could set up some basic rules of etiquette regarding its use. What follows is a general guide that anyone can use to be more civilized when using mobile phones.

The first basic rule is that when you are in a public place or in the company of people you consider important, turn the ringer on your phone off. Phones now have voice mail, and you'll be well served by eliminating interruptions. If you absolutely must take a call, set the phone on vibrate and politely excuse yourself to answer the call.

If you cannot avoid taking a call in a public place, keep the conversation short and quiet. With the new digital phones, you can speak softly and still be heard. Be mindful of how annoying it is for others to have to listen to a long one-sided phone conversation.

If you find yourself driving and talking on the phone, realize that it might be safer to pull over to finish the call. Alternatively, purchase a hands-free unit for your phone. Statistics show that talking on a cell phone while driving is just as dangerous as driving drunk.

SHAKING HANDS

There was a time when deals were sealed with a handshake. Nowadays, the handshake is an important component in that very powerful first impression. The moment you are being introduced to someone, or when the prospective employer is a few feet away from you, extend your right hand. A firm handshake is best. Remember, you want the person you are meeting to know that you are a solid person who can be trusted and counted on. On the flip side, do not injure the person you are meeting. You want to make the person feel good. Figure 35 shows two examples of incorrect handshakes followed by the correct form.

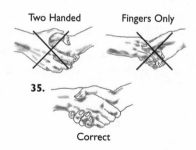

Two Handed Fingers Only

35.

Correct

When the opportunity presents itself, square your shoulders to the person you want to greet. Smile, look the person in the eye, and extend your right hand. Your fingers should be relatively close to each other, but not actually touching, and your thumb should be pointed straight up. As your hand meets the other hand, make sure you try to touch your thumb-finger web to that of the other person. Next, place your thumb on his or her hand, and squeeze the hand as if you were squeezing the ketchup out of a plastic container. You should shake for about three pumps, then slowly pull your hand away.

Nametags should be worn on the right breast pocket to make it easier for others to read your name when you shake their hands. When you are standing at a cocktail party, be sure to keep your drink in your left hand. Since you will shake with your right hand, you do not want it to be cold and wet from the glass. If you shake someone's hand and find theirs to be wet, cold, or sweaty, do not draw attention to the condition, even in a joking manner. Act as if it were completely normal and move on. By politely ignoring it, you will help the other person feel accepted and consequently more comfortable with you.

As odd as it sounds, you should practice shaking hands with family members or friends. Your goal is to let the other person know that you have a strong handshake but not to break every bone in his or her hand. With a good handshake you will present a strong first impression and again illustrate your attention to detail.

TABLE MANNERS

Any discussion of professional conduct would be incomplete without a discussion of table manners. Many professional meetings begin, include, or conclude with a meal. While good manners may not explicitly help you, bad manners will definitely hurt you.

To get your bearings, see the illustration of a typical table setting in figure 36. The simplest rule for using silverware is to work from the outside in toward the plate as the meal progresses. Your forks are on the left. If there are two, the smaller, outside fork is the salad fork, and the larger, inner one is your dinner fork. On the right, from the outside, is your spoon and knife with its blade facing toward the plate. There may also be a soupspoon. A spoon or fork found above your plate is for dessert and your beverage and coffee cup will be located on the upper right corner of your table setting. Your salad plate will be on your left side with your bread plate.

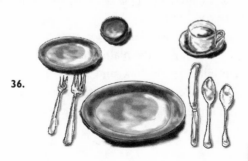

36.

As soon as you sit down at the table with others, find your napkin, unfold it, and put it on your lap. Next, leave your nondominant hand on your lap or on the edge of the table and keep it there for most of the meal. You will want to eat with your dominant hand. The only time you will use both hands is to cut your food. To cut properly, hold your fork upside down with your nondominant hand and your knife with your dominant hand. As soon as you have finished cutting, place the knife back on the right side of the plate or across the top of the plate, and switch your fork to your dominant hand to eat.

When eating bread, break off a small piece, butter it, and eat it. Do not butter the whole piece of bread or roll all at once. Also, do not cut your food into many pieces. Simply cut off the piece you will eat, chew it well, and then cut again. Use your napkin often to clean any crumbs or food pieces from your lips. When someone asks you to pass the salt or pepper, pass the salt and pepper at the same time. Never reach across anyone's "personal space." Simply ask them to pass the item to you or pass it to them to pass farther down the table.

If you get up during the meal, place the napkin on your chair. This lets the wait staff know that you will be returning soon. When you finish with a spoon, place it on the saucer under your soup dish or coffee cup, not in the bowl or cup itself.

As soon as you have finished your meal, place your knife across the top of the plate, with the blade facing you. Next place your fork and other used utensils closer to the middle of the plate, tines down, and parallel to the knife. As soon as you complete your meal, use your napkin, fold it loosely, and place it on the table (figure 37). If you follow these simple rules, you will greatly lessen the chances of committing a serious faux pas at a business meal.

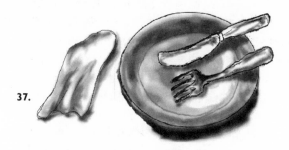

37.

Paying for meals is often a confusing element of etiquette, but there are generally accepted rules you can follow. First, when you are being interviewed for a job or your boss is taking you out for a performance review, you can expect them to pay for the meal.

The most basic rule is that the person who invites the other for the meal usually pays for it. The next rule for paying is that if there is ever a question, take the whole bill yourself and treat the others to a nice meal. By paying most of the time, you gain several advantages over those with whom you eat. First, there is an inherent belief that if you pay, others are somewhat indebted to you. Second, by paying, you eliminate the awkwardness of waiting for someone to pick up the tab.

For most businesses, when eating with clients, you should plan to pay for the meal. If they do take the bill, be sure to get it next time and at least alternate paying. You should avoid letting your clients pay for too many of your meals.

Usually you will not be eating with your superiors on a regular basis, so it is acceptable for them to pay for the meal. But, if you do usually eat with them, you should expect to pay for yourself most of the time. One caveat is if you invite the superior to eat for a special purpose, like to ask for a special raise or promotion, you should try to pay.

Much like eating with superiors, you probably will not eat with your subordinates very often. Make a point to pay for their meals some of the time, but do not pay every time, as they may begin to expect it. When eating with those at your level, you should usually pay your own way, but pick up the check every once in a while for a nice treat.

If you are in sales, or usually take your clients out to lunch or dinner, following these tips can help you and your career. When you invite someone to eat, you are making a big impression. Unfortunately, just asking someone to eat does not necessarily mean that it will be a good impression.

The best way to prepare yourself for good impressions is to build relationships with local restaurants near your office and around town. Pick three or four that serve a variety of foods, and one or two with a special theme or menu. You should make a point to visit these places at least once a month. Tip very well (25–30 percent) and be friendly with the host or hostess and servers. After a few visits, ask them to give you an account. They can either bill you at the end of each month or keep your credit card on file and charge all your meals to it. Either way, be sure that many of the servers and host know who you are and treat you with respect.

This relationship allows you to focus on the business at hand, knowing that you will have great service and that the bill is not an issue. Other benefits of having a relationship with a restaurant are that it will help get you a great table on short notice, you will not have to wait to be seated, and you will get excellent service.

Once you have your relationships firmly in place, you will have more flexibility when making plans with your clients. Ask them where they will be before you plan to eat and cater the invitation to your client's location. This will also give you a bit of an edge with the client in the meetings by having a comfortable environment for your meals. You can avoid many of the hassles that spring up when eating out. The question of paying for the meal will be answered as soon as you sit at your table, your drink will be waiting for you, and the staff will address you by name. Your clients will also be impressed with your good rapport with the staff and your excellent attention to detail.

WRITING A RÉSUMÉ 23

A good résumé can help you land the job of your dreams. A bad résumé can ensure that you will not get the job. This chapter will provide some basic tips that can really help you promote yourself through your résumé. The first and most important thing is to be honest. Aside from the obvious moral problems involved with lying, there are numerous other reasons to be honest. For those of you who might be tempted to lie or "embellish" your résumé, pay attention and you will quickly see why you should not.

Interviewers and human resources (HR) professionals are, by their nature, detectives. Most examine every detail with a suspicious eye and are trained to look for lies. Let's be clear: If you lie on your résumé and get caught (and you will eventually be caught), you will not get the job, or worse, you will be subsequently fired after the truth is known. Plus, people will talk. When the word gets out that you are dishonest, your career is over and you will not be respected. It is as simple as that.

At the same time, it is important not to be modest. Your résumé is your best, and maybe your only, chance to "toot your own horn." Tell prospective employers the good things you have done. If you have accomplished

John Q. Doe

Home address   School address
Anytown, USA   Collegetown, USA
Home phone   School phone
Home e-mail   School e-mail

OBJECTIVE: To obtain employment at a major public accounting firm.

EDUCATION: **State University**, Class of 2002 Collegetown, USA
Accounting and Finance Major, GPA of 3.4 1998–2002
Honors Society, Dean's List Spring 1999

Central High School, Class of 1998 Anytown, USA
Honors in Math, Science and History 1994–1998
Lettered in Football and Baseball

EMPLOYMENT: **Dewey, Cheatam, and Howe, CPA** Anytown, USA
Summer Intern in Audit Department Summer 2000
Learned MS Office and Quickbooks Software

Acme Products, Sales Division Anytown, USA
Sold household products door to door Summer 1999

Tasty Freeze Ice Cream Anytown, USA
Store Manager Summer 1998

HOBBIES: **Umpire for Little League** Anytown, USA
Volunteer Umpire for Local Little League 1997–Present

Reading for the Blind Anytown, USA
Read School Books for Blind Children 1999–Present

something special, talk about it. If you were not the valedictorian, the captain of the football team, or a national merit scholar, you may think you have nothing to say, but that is rarely true. Simply look back on the last few years and find the things you did that will make you marketable in the job market.

Set up a résumé in the following format. Begin with your full name, centered across the top. Use a font size slightly larger than that of the body of the résumé. If you have one address, center it below your name and include your phone number and e-mail address. If you have two addresses—for example if you are in college and live away from home—list both, justifying one right and the other left. Again, include phone numbers and e-mail addresses with both.

In discussing addresses and phone numbers, one word of caution must be included. Be careful about using your current employer's address, phone numbers, or e-mail address on your résumé. Unless you are certain that your current employer will not mind that you are looking for a new job, use only your home address, phone number, and e-mail address. Having said that, be sure you have an answering machine or voice-mail at your home. Also, remember that your potential employer will hear your message, so be certain that it is professional, short, and to the point. Try something like, "Hello. You have reached <first and last name>. I'm sorry I cannot take your call now, but if you would please leave your name and telephone number, I will return your call as soon as possible."

Below your name, address, phone number, and e-mail address at the top of the page, you should insert a line separating this information from the body of the résumé.

State your employment objective clearly and professionally. For example, "To obtain full-time employment with a major public accounting firm." If your actual objective is unclear, or you do not feel comfortable including one, do not use one. Keep in mind that you may change objectives and items on the resume to conform to each job for which you are applying.

The education section of your résumé should come next if you are right out of school. If you have been in the professional world for more than a year, you might choose to place the employment section first. Base your decision on what you think is the most relevant element of your recent past.

Depending on the last level of education you completed, you may include or exclude high school data. (If you have your Ph.D., high school information will probably not interest your employers.) If you are a recent college graduate, you probably want to include your high school name, your GPA, any honors you received, sports you played, and activities in which you were involved. Be smart. If you did well, say so. If you were not a star student, do not say anything. Build up your strengths, and avoid your weaknesses. To the far right of this information, include the years you were in school, as well as the location of each.

Experience or employment history usually comes next. Here you want to focus on your accomplishments, showing the jobs you have had and how they relate to your objective, a prospective position, or your potential employer's business.

The final section can include your hobbies, interests, and involvement in outside groups and organizations. Remember that what you include on your résumé is up to you. If you feel that the inclusion or exclusion of any item is justified and will help a potential employer make a decision in your favor, go for it. Keep your résumé condensed and to the point. If you are new to the job world, try to keep it to just one page.

INTERVIEWING

When you obtain an appointment for an interview with a prospective employer, learn about the company and the job for which you are applying before the interview takes place. The Internet is a great place to start, but company newsletters, annual reports, and magazine articles also can be helpful.

Try to gain a general understanding of the company as if you were going to write a report about it. Find out who the top officers are and, if possible, their personality types. Almost without exception, the leader's personality is indicative of the corporate culture. Also study current events involving the company and its industry. You can be sure that most topics in the news will be fair game for the interviewer's questions. Current events will also give you a good base for questions to ask.

Arrive to the interview a few minutes early, in your most professional attire. Once the interview starts, you will have a few moments to get a feel for the interviewer. Build rapport with him or her by sitting up straight, smiling softly, and looking him or her in the eyes when you speak. The first few minutes will create the interviewer's basic impression of you, and quite possibly, affect your chances of getting hired. Often he or she will begin the interview by discussing your résumé or an employment form designed by their company. Since the information will be familiar to you, this will help you relax. As discussed earlier in the résumé section, you must be honest. If you lie, you will be uncomfortable and stressed during the interview instead of being relaxed and freely discussing your accomplishments. Be modest, but positive about your experiences and be sure to be able to explain how you overcame problems or hurdles in your life. Most interviewers now ask you for a situation in which you dealt with difficulty or failure, and what you learned in the process.

If you were previously employed, the interviewer will almost always ask about your former employer. Do not take this as an invitation to complain about how horrible your experience was or how much you hate your old boss, even if it is true. This question is designed to evaluate what kind of relationship you had with your previous employer. Be sure to be honest, but do not say that your boss hated you or that you hated him or her. Try to mention the benefits of working at that job and what you learned there that will help you in your next position.

One of the biggest fears of candidates is that they may have to answer difficult questions. In general, if you are faced with a question that you cannot solve, do not guess or make up an answer. It is much easier to say "I don't know, but I will find out and call you with the answer tomorrow." You will appear much more intelligent and honest, and you will not have to be afraid of the truth.

You may face some minor obstacles in your interview. The worst of these is the question from your interviewer that seems off the wall. He or she may call it a "probing" or "character" question. These are supposed to give the interviewer some sort of insight into what kind of person you are. A good example of this would be "If you could be any kind of fruit, what kind would you be?" If you are asked a question like this, do your best to answer it, but do not stress about it too much.

You may be asked a question designed to test your analytical and problem-solving abilities. This could be a system question or a riddle. A system question tests your system in attempting to solve a problem. For example, let's say your interviewer asks, "How many gas stations are there in the United States?" He or she is interested not in the exact amount of gas sold but in your system that brings you to an answer. He or she will test your assumptions and math for logic, not necessarily numerical accuracy.

Answer this type of question by thinking it through. For example, count the number of gas stations in your town and estimate the population. Divide your population by that of the United States. Using ratios, now divide the number of stations by the percentage of your town's population and you will have a rough, but good, answer.

The interviewer may ask you a complex riddle that requires you to think "outside of the box." Knowing how to answer these questions can be very helpful, especially if you have seen the question before. There are several good books on riddles that will give you some samples and some tips on solving new problems. Another good bet is to talk to others who have recently interviewed with the company and ask them for some pointers. Since each company is a bit different, it helps to have some insight into the nuances of each company before you get there.

Often in the interview process, you will be invited to a lunch. It will either be as part of a full day of interviews or just for a "relaxed" setting. Do not be fooled; this setting is no more relaxing than being in an office. It does, however, give the employer a great chance to see you outside of the office, and it serves as a window to the "true you." You are always under the microscope, even at lunch. Watch how you treat others, especially the staff at the restaurant.

You might think that because the interviewer is going to pick up the check (and he or she will), you can order anything you want. This is not, however, an invitation for you to order the most expensive item on the menu. Choose a meal with a moderate price and one that is easy to eat. That basically means avoiding finger foods and pasta dishes that can really make a mess. You want the interviewer to focus on your ability to work well, not on the huge bill and the sauce on your shirt.

A simple test that IBM used in the 1970s was called "The Salt Test." They would check to see if the candidate would salt or pepper his or her food before tasting it. They surmised that anyone who would salt their food before tasting it was too quick to judge and thus was not IBM material. Although this may seem to be an insane test, realize that some interviewers still use this test. So, even if you love your salt or pepper, make sure you taste your food first. It's pretty easy to do, and it could save you from making a huge mistake.

At the end of every interview, you will be given an opportunity to ask questions. Use it. Find out what you want to know but have not been able to learn from your initial research. Having said that, there is such a thing as a stupid question in an interview situation. This can include asking how much money the position pays, what the vacation policy is, what the company does, and what your chances of getting the job are. Make a point to ask something that will help you to be chosen above other candidates. Ask about a "day in the life" of the person currently in the position for which you are applying or how the company can offer you growth, both personally and professionally. Depending on the interviewer's perceived receptivity for suggestions, you might want to use your earlier research on the company to make a suggestion for a new opportunity they might consider. Many companies would appreciate this initiative.

After the interview, be sure to follow up with a thank-you letter to the interviewer or interviewers. This can take the form of a card or letter but not e-mail. The most important part is to thank the individual for his or her time and consideration. You may also answer questions you were unable to answer during the interview, provide other information, or ask another question. Be sure to personalize the communication by making a reference to your interview. If you meet with more than one person, be sure to send a separate thank-you letter to each.

BEING ON TIME AND ORGANIZED 25

Not everyone finds being on time easy. Most people who arrive on time and call when they say they will, have to work at it. Professionals must become masters of time. Making a point of being exactly on time is an obvious way of showing your attention to detail. People who are known for punctuality are also well respected and trusted.

When arriving for a meeting, show up about one minute before the scheduled time of the meeting. You do not want to rush someone by showing up well before your set time. On the other hand, being late shows a lack of consideration. If you become unavoidably detained, call. That is what mobile phones are for. Realize, however, that you should make every effort to be on time. The first time you plan to meet someone at an unfamiliar location—or if you are concerned about being late—plan on arriving 15 to 20 minutes early. You can use this extra time in your car or outside the building to deal with small administrative tasks.

The key to good organization is planning, so get a good planner. Many different styles are available, and as long as you will use it, the type does not matter. First, make sure that your planner allows you to plan on a daily, weekly, monthly, and long-term basis. It should have room for names, addresses, and phone numbers. Some even have clear plastic sheets that can hold about six business cards per page. Keep the cards you use most in these pages. For the others that you accumulate, you should consider getting a three-ring binder with ten-card sheets as previously mentioned. This will allow you to keep your business cards in an accessible, portable form.

BUSINESS COMMUNICATION 26

A business letter is an important part of professional communication. By following the proper format, you will illustrate to the recipient your knowledge of business culture and get your message across effectively. It is best if you justify all type on the left. Begin your letter with the date, followed by the name and address of the individual to whom you are writing. Next, greet the reader by the name you commonly use in conversation. If you have not met, do not use their first name. Make the letter as clear, straightforward, and easy to read as possible. In the first or second sentence, convey the purpose of writing, and spend the rest of the letter discussing the point. Do your best to keep the letter to one page; 95 percent of all of your communications should be limited to one page only. Single-space the type but include an extra space between paragraphs. You may or may not indent the first line of each paragraph: it is a matter of personal style. When you complete the body of the text, conclude with "Sincerely," or "Best regards." Leave a few spaces for your signature, then type your full name below.

MEMORANDUM

DATE: October 23, 2000
TO: All Employees
FROM: John Q. Doe, HR Director   *JQD*
RE: Halloween Party

After several months of meetings and employee surveys, the human resources department has decided to host our annual Halloween Party in the office on Halloween afternoon.

The entire day of Halloween will be a casual day for those of you who wish to dress up in a festive costume. Refreshments will be provided, but we ask that you each bring a bag of candy for needy children.

Any questions may be forwarded to me via voice mail at x1040 or e-mail.

The proper format for a business memo is constantly changing, but the following is a basic template. First, type a capitalized "MEMORANDUM" to signify the format.

Justifying all type on the left, begin with the date, and then skip a few lines. Type "To:" and identify the recipient by his or her complete name. Next, type "From:" and follow with your full name. Below the names, type "Re:" or "Subj:" and indicate the reason for your communication. This should be three or four words describing the memo. Then write your paragraphs as separate groups, without indenting the first line. No conclusion is necessary, and again, keep it to one page. After you have printed the memorandum, initial it to the right of your name.

E-mail and voice mail are growing in popularity since most offices use both as communicating tools. Although these formats are informal, remember that you are a professional and need to conduct yourself as one. Begin your e-mails with the proper salutation, use professional language, and keep them short. In a voice mail, greet the person, convey your point clearly, and keep the message short. Most voice mail systems allow you to erase and rerecord your message if you make a mistake. Take advantage of this option; you always want to sound the best you can. This may mean taking extra time to learn the system, and the functions it performs.

In the course of a long business day, there are many things we can't seem to get done. This happens to everyone and is understandable. There are some things, however, that you must do. Returning phone calls, even those you do not want to, is one of the things you must do every day. By being one of the few professionals who returns all phone calls, you will set yourself above the many people in business who think (incorrectly) that they are too busy to return phone calls.

Because so much of business is done over the phone, it is important to develop good phone skills. Make sure you speak clearly and at a moderate pace. Smile when you speak, and be cordial. Many professionals now never meet their clients face-to-face; the phone is their only link. For these people, a professional phone voice and demeanor are incredibly important. Ask your family, friends, and coworkers to listen to how you sound on the phone, to be sure you are making the proper impression.

The language you use in the professional world is important; an extensive vocabulary can quickly illustrate your intelligence and creativity. At the same time, there is no excuse for swearing in the office. It might seem cool and part of being a big shot, but no gentleman swears in the workplace. The extensive use of four-letter words shows complete incompetence in the use of the English language and is characteristic of someone who is inconsiderate to his coworkers and clients. If you must express your disdain, show your intelligence and creativity and use some more descriptive words.

Learn a valuable lesson from cartoons and movies geared toward children. Listen to the way supervillains express their anger and pick your favorite. Some of the better ones are "rats," "blast," and "gadzooks!" It is your responsibility to contain your anger and use suitable terms.

If you can change this element of your conduct and use silly terms, you will do two valuable things. First, you will show your colleagues and clients that you respect them enough not to swear in front of them. Second, you also stand a pretty good chance of getting them to laugh and see your humorous side when you say "blast"! By working to stop swearing and better express yourself in the professional setting, you will help enhance your image among your coworkers and clients.

E-MAIL PRIVACY 27

E-mail is now a common form of communication in most workplaces. Many employees connect to the Internet and communicate with friends and family all over the world on company time. Some employers condone this, others do not. Be sure to check your company's policy regarding personal e-mails during working hours before unnecessarily endangering your job. The problem arises when employees believe that the messages they send are private. By law, every e-mail you send and receive at work can be read by your employer. It is unclear how many companies check messages, but the important point is that the possibility exists. When using e-mail at work, assume that your boss and everyone else will read every word you write.

If you feel the need to send personal e-mails, establish a personal account through an Internet Service Provider. There are also several free e-mail services on the Internet. Realize that the same laws exist for surfing the Internet and visiting the Web. Any employer can get a listing of every Web site you visited when using your employer's system, so be careful. If you do visit sites that you would not want the entire office to know about, surf the Net away from work. Also, be sparing in your non-business use of the Internet. Your employer can track the time you spend and locations you visit on the Web, and this could definitely be a career-limiting move.

OFFICE POLITICS

28

"People will talk." You have heard it before, but now at work, it is much more prevalent. When you finally get your job, you will find that office politics and the proverbial "grapevine" not only exist but often run rampant. You must be prepared for this; expect it and accept it. Unfortunately, it is human nature.

Having said this, do not play the game. It is very easy to sit with your coworkers and complain about your boss, other coworkers, or subordinates. Do not do it. There are no good reasons to sit in on these discussions, let alone participate in them. The information—or misinformation—is harmful not only to the subjects of the discussion but to the speaker and the listener as well. By participating, you often gather faulty information. Think about it. If you tell others how you dislike someone with whom you are usually pleasant, they will realize that they cannot trust anything you say. Rise above gossip. Stick to your work and the tasks that will help you succeed. You will be stronger for it in the end.

When you work to develop a friendly rapport with your coworkers, be smart about it. A proven plan is to be respectful with everyone and give possible friendships plenty of time to develop. People respond well when they are treated with respect. Most office friendships are best developed slowly. If you make your coworkers feel comfortable by treating them with respect, you will build strong relationships over time.

When first building relationships, be wary of constantly going out after work with your new coworkers. A drink or two after work is usually a very good idea, but keep it to one or two. The key to after-hours socialization is to limit its time and extent. Becoming too friendly too soon often results in an awkward relationship that may turn ugly. There are several benefits to getting to know your fellow workers out of the office, just remember to give the relationships time to develop. Along the same vein, be extremely careful when dating someone from the office. Intraoffice romances usually end badly and can destroy careers.

When in the office, or even in an after-hours social setting, act as if every action you take is being recorded. Yes, this is a cynical view, but it is the safe course of action. Refrain from making lewd jokes, because they will almost certainly offend someone. Similarly, do not imitate someone who stutters or has an accent. This will almost always get back to the person you are imitating and definitely harm you. Even if you think you are funny, you are still rude and out of line. Remember, if you treat everyone with respect, you will build strong relationships with your coworkers.

Most of us grew up in an environment where guys were physical with each other. In the locker room, guys may have punched each other on the arm in a friendly manner. On the ball field, coaches pat the players on their backsides. The reality is that any touching, of either men or women, is inappropriate for the professional environment.

The exponential increase in sexual harassment cases proves this point well. Although it is somewhat awkward, when you work in the professional setting, you must avoid physical contact with your coworkers. It illustrates your respect for the person's "personal space," as well as your professionalism. By simply treating your coworkers with respect, you will immediately show your exemplary professional conduct.

Remember that current-events class we took in fifth grade? The homework was to watch the news on television or read the paper and stay informed. Today, similarly, part of your professional conduct requires you to stay informed of the issues currently facing the world.

The Internet is full of sites that provide quick and clear news to help you stay informed. Look at www.cnn.com, www.yahoo.com, and www.cnbc.com.

There is an obvious need to stay informed about current events affecting your company, profession, and industry. If your biggest competitor files for bankruptcy, it is important for you to have a basic knowledge about what happened and what the impact might be on you and your company.

What about general current events? Do you really need to stay informed about civil rights in a foreign land? The answer is yes. There are many things you can learn by keeping up to date with current events. But more importantly, people are often judged by their ability to engage in small talk. It is imperative to be able to speak intelligently with your coworkers.

Although you may not care, most professionals need to have at least a rudimentary knowledge of the issues facing the world today. The reason for this is that in many of the "relaxed professional settings" when small talk is prevalent, the discussion topics often turn to current events. It is quite embarrassing when your boss asks you a question about your thoughts on a new political issue, and you have no idea what it is, let alone what you think of it.

Remember that current events will come up in daily conversations, and it pays to have some knowledge about them. You are constantly being judged; by keeping up to date, you can really show off your attention to detail.

CONCLUSION

With the simple techniques discussed in this book, you can begin to take command of your appearance and professional demeanor. People will notice your attention to detail and understand that you care about your appearance and professional reputation. If you keep your appearance in order and act like a gentleman, you will probably find that you are treated with respect. But most importantly, you will also feel more comfortable about yourself and be able to do your best work. Remember, attention to detail can be a great help to your career and your life.

If you would like to stay informed about seasonal trends and developments, fill out the form in the back of the book for a FREE one-year subscription to the *Attention to Detail* newsletter.

If you have any thoughts, ideas, suggestions, questions, or comments, please send them to: *Attention to Detail* Newsletter, Greenleaf Enterprises, 660 Elmwood Point, Aurora, Ohio 44202. You can also call us at (800) 932-5420. Visit our Web site at *www.greenleafenterprises.com*, or send an e-mail to: *email@greenleafenterprises.com*.

SELECTED BIBLIOGRAPHY

Bridges, John. *How to Be a Gentleman*. Nashville, TN: Rutledge Hill Press, 1998.

Davis, Jeannie. *Beyond Hello*. Denver, CO: Now Hear This Publishing, 1999.

Flusser, Alan. *Style and the Man*. New York, NY: HarperStyle, 1996.

Friedman, Steve. *The Gentleman's Guide to Life*. New York, NY: Three Rivers Press, 1997.

Grant, Lynella. *The Business Card Book*. Tucson, AZ: Off the Page Press, 1998.

Greenleaf, Clinton T., III. *Attention to Detail: A Gentleman's Guide to Professional Appearance and Conduct*. Cleveland, OH: Greenleaf Enterprises, Inc., 1998.

Greenleaf, Clinton T., III, and Stefani Schaefer. *Attention to Detail: A Woman's Guide to Professional Appearance and Conduct*. Cleveland, OH: Greenleaf Enterprises, Inc., 1999.

Gross, Kim Johnson. *Men's Wardrobe (Chic Simple)*, New York, NY: Knopf, 1998.

Karlen, Josh, and Christopher Sulavik. *The Indispensable Guide to Classic Men's Clothing*. New York, NY: Tatra Press, 1999.

Meehan, Tim. *Suit Yourself*. Birmingham, AL: J. T. Meehan Publishing, 1999.

Omelanuk, Scott, and Ted Allen. *Esquire's Things a Man Should Know About Style*. New York, NY: Riverhead Books, 1999.

Waldrop, Dawn E. *Best Impressions*. Cleveland, OH: Best Impressions, 1997.

About the Author

Clint Greenleaf is Chairman and CEO of Greenleaf Enterprises, Inc., and Greenleaf Book Group LLC. He spent three years training in the United States Marine Corps ROTC program before graduating with a B.A. in economics/accounting from the College of the Holy Cross in Worcester, Massachusetts. While in college, he worked as an admissions officer, interviewing high school seniors for entry into the school, where he noticed a need for such a book. After graduation, he worked at Deloitte & Touche, a "Big 5" accounting firm, and passed the CPA exam.

Greenleaf Enterprises

For more information on professional appearance and conduct, as well as a resource guide and information on ordering items like shoetrees and other products, visit *www.greenleafenterprises.com* or call (800) 932-5420 to order a catalog.

INDEX

The Everything® Etiquette Book

Nat Segaloff

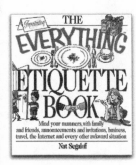

Trade paperback, $12.95
ISBN: 1-55850-807-4

Most people think of etiquette as a collection of silly rules which snobbish people use to make everybody else feel out of place. Well, not anymore! *The Everything® Etiquette Book* gives you the comprehensive resource you need to deal with every conceivable situation you might encounter. With great advice on everything from neighborly behavior to office protocol, and from making new friends to keeping the peace in your family, this book will help you put your best foot forward. This single volume distills hundreds of years of proper behavior into streamlined rules you can apply to today's world. It features quick tips and helpful hints that you can apply every day.